Eating to Lower Your High Blood Cholesterol

**National Institutes of Health
U.S. Public Health Service**

Fredonia Books
Amsterdam, The Netherlands

Eating to Lower Your High Blood Cholesterol

by
National Institutes of Health
U.S. Public Health Service

ISBN: 1-4101-0903-8

Copyright © 2006 by Fredonia Books

Reprinted from the 1989 edition

Fredonia Books
Amsterdam, The Netherlands
http://www.fredoniabooks.com

All rights reserved, including the right to reproduce this book, or portions thereof, in any form.

Table of Contents

Eating to Lower Your High Blood Cholesterol   1

What You Need to Know About High Blood Cholesterol   2
Why Should You Know Your Blood Cholesterol Level?   2
How High Is Your Blood Cholesterol Level?   2
What Should Your Blood Cholesterol Goal Be?   4
How Does Your Blood Cholesterol Become High?   4

The Recommended Treatment: A Blood Cholesterol-Lowering Diet   5
What Changes Should You Make in Your Diet?   5
    Eat Less High-Fat Food   5
    Eat Less Saturated Fat   6
    Substitute Unsaturated Fat for Saturated Fat   7
    Eat Less High-Cholesterol Food   8
    Substitute Complex Carbohydrates for Saturated Fat   8
    Maintain a Desirable Weight   9
How Should You Change Your Daily Menu?   9
What Kind of Success Can You Expect?   13

How to Change Your Eating Patterns   14
Shop for Foods That Are Low in Saturated Fat and Cholesterol   14
Read the Labels   22
Low-Fat Cooking Tips   23
Where Can You Go For Help?   25

Glossary   27

List of Appendices

Appendix 1:	Desirable Weights for Men and Women	31
Appendix 2:	Meats	32
Appendix 3:	Poultry	37
Appendix 4:	Fish and Shellfish	39
Appendix 5:	Dairy Products	41
Appendix 6:	Frozen Desserts	43
Appendix 7:	Fats and Oils	44
Appendix 8:	Nuts and Seeds	45
Appendix 9:	Breads, Cereals, Pasta, Rice, and Dried Peas and Beans	46
Appendix 10:	Sweets and Snacks	48
Appendix 11:	Miscellaneous	50
	A Guide to Choosing Low-Saturated Fat, Low-Cholesterol Foods	54

Eating to Lower Your High Blood Cholesterol

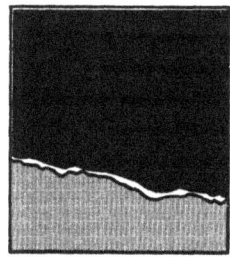

High blood cholesterol is a serious problem. Along with high blood pressure and cigarette smoking, it is one of the three major modifiable risk factors for coronary heart disease. Approximately 25 percent of the adult population 20 years of age and older has "high" blood cholesterol levels–levels that are high enough to need intensive medical attention. More than half of all adult Americans have a blood cholesterol level that is higher than "desirable."

Because high blood cholesterol is a risk to your health, you need to take steps to lower your blood cholesterol level. The best way to do this is to make sure you eat foods that are low in saturated fat and cholesterol. The purpose of this brochure is to help you learn how to choose these foods. This brochure will also introduce you to key concepts about blood cholesterol and its relationship to your diet. For example, it includes basic (but very important) information about saturated fat–the dietary component most responsible for raising blood cholesterol—and about dietary cholesterol–the cholesterol contained in food.

This brochure is divided into three parts. The first part of the brochure gives background information about high blood cholesterol and its relationship to heart disease. The second part introduces key points on diet changes and better food choices to lower blood cholesterol levels.

Finally, in the third part more specific instructions are given for modifying eating patterns to lower your blood cholesterol, choosing low-saturated fat and low-cholesterol foods, and preparing low-fat dishes.

The "glossary" provides easy definitions of new or unfamiliar terms. The "appendices" that follow the glossary list the saturated fat and cholesterol content of a variety of foods.

What You Need to Know About High Blood Cholesterol

Why Should You Know Your Blood Cholesterol Level?

There are important reasons for you to be concerned about your blood cholesterol level. Over time, cholesterol, fat, and other substances can build up in the walls of your arteries (a process called *atherosclerosis*) and can slow or block the flow of blood to your heart. Among many things, blood carries a constant supply of oxygen to the heart. Without oxygen, heart muscle weakens, resulting in chest pain, heart attacks, or even death. However, for many people there are no warning symptoms or signs until late in the disease process.

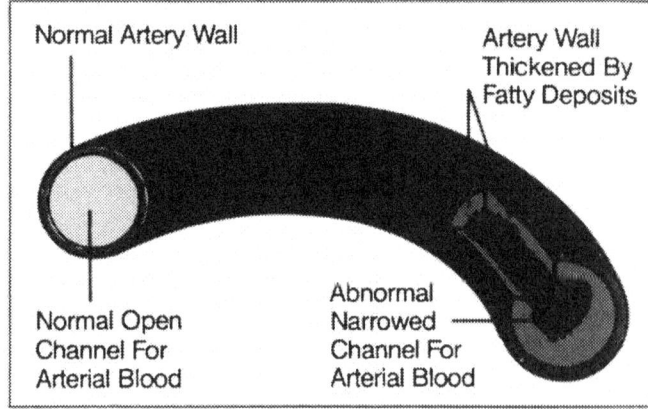

Heart disease is the leading cause of death in this country. Scientists have known for a long time that high blood cholesterol, high blood pressure, and smoking all increase the risk of heart disease.

Research now shows that the risk of developing atherosclerosis or coronary heart disease also increases as the blood cholesterol level increases. And it has now been proven that lowering high blood cholesterol, like controlling high blood pressure and avoiding smoking, will reduce this risk.

How High Is Your Blood Cholesterol Level?

The medical community recently set guidelines for classifying blood cholesterol levels. They advise that a total cholesterol level less than 200 mg/dl is **"desirable"** for adults - above 200 mg/dl the risk of coronary heart disease steadily increases. The classifications of total blood cholesterol in the following chart are related to the risk of developing heart disease.

Does Your Total Blood Cholesterol Level Increase Your Risk For Developing Coronary Heart Disease?

Desirable Blood Cholesterol	Borderline-High Blood Cholesterol	High Blood Cholesterol
Less than 200 mg/dl	200-239 mg/dl	240 mg/dl and above

If your total cholesterol level is in the range of 200-239 mg/dl, you are classified as having **"borderline-high"** blood cholesterol and are at increased risk for coronary heart disease compared to those with lower levels. However, if you have no other factors that increase your risk for coronary heart disease,* you should not need intensive medical attention. But you should make dietary changes to lower your level and thus reduce your risk of coronary heart disease.

On the other hand, if you have borderline-high blood cholesterol and have coronary heart disease or two other risk factors for coronary heart disease, you need special medical attention. In fact, you should be treated in the same way as people with **"high"** blood cholesterol – 240 mg/dl or greater – who could be at high risk for developing coronary heart disease and warrant more detailed evaluation and medical treatment.

Additional evaluation helps your physician determine more accurately your risk of coronary heart disease and make decisions about your treatment. Specifically, your doctor will probably want to measure your low density lipoprotein (LDL) cholesterol level – since LDL-cholesterol more accurately reflects your risk for coronary heart disease than a total cholesterol level alone. LDL-cholesterol levels of 130 mg/dl or greater increase your risk for developing coronary heart disease. After evaluating your LDL-cholesterol level and other risk factors for coronary heart disease, your physician will determine your treatment program.

Remember: *As your cholesterol level rises, your risk of developing coronary heart disease increases.*

*Risk factors for coronary heart disease include high blood pressure, cigarette smoking, family history of coronary heart disease before the age of 55, diabetes, vascular disease, obesity, and being male.

What Should Your Blood Cholesterol Goal Be?

If you have high blood cholesterol or need intensive treatment because of other risk factors, your physician will probably set an LDL-cholesterol goal for you. This goal will vary depending on your overall risk and what may be a realistic goal for you. Remember, a total cholesterol level below 200 mg/dl and an LDL-cholesterol level below 130 mg/dl are desirable. Even though achieving your LDL-cholesterol goal is more important than your total cholesterol goal, your physician may choose to check your progress by measuring your total cholesterol level because it is a good deal simpler and you do not have to fast before its measurement. When you reach your total cholesterol goal, your physician will probably measure your LDL-cholesterol to confirm that you also reached your LDL-cholesterol goal.

How Does Your Blood Cholesterol Level Become High?

What you eat can raise or lower your blood cholesterol level. The average American diet of high-saturated fat, high-cholesterol foods like fatty meats, many dairy products, fried foods, cookies, cakes, and eggs contributes to high blood cholesterol.

In some countries like Japan, for example, people eat diets rich in rice, fruits, vegetables, and fish. The Japanese have lower blood cholesterol levels and lower rates of coronary heart disease than Americans. This is in part because these foods are low in fat, particularly saturated fat, which is the greatest **dietary contributor** to high blood cholesterol.

While diet plays an important role in raising or lowering your blood cholesterol level, **inherited tendencies** also influence your level. A small percentage of people can eat a diet that is high in saturated fat and cholesterol and still maintain a low blood cholesterol level. On the other hand, there is a small percentage of people who may not be able to lower their blood cholesterol even with a low-saturated fat, low-cholesterol diet. However, both of these groups constitute a minority of the population of the United States. Most people can control their blood cholesterol levels by following a diet that is low in saturated fat and cholesterol.

The Recommended Treatment: A Blood Cholesterol-Lowering Diet

Whatever the reasons may be for your high blood cholesterol level – diet, heredity, or both – the treatment your doctor will prescribe first is a diet. If your blood cholesterol level has not decreased sufficiently after carefully following the diet for 6 months, your doctor may consider adding cholesterol-lowering medication to your dietary treatment. Remember, diet is a very essential step in the treatment of high blood cholesterol. Cholesterol-lowering medications are more effective when combined with diet. Thus they are meant to supplement, not replace, a low-saturated fat, low-cholesterol diet.

What Changes Should You Make in Your Diet?

The following chart illustrates some guidelines for dietary changes to help you lower your blood cholesterol level. Your new diet is low in saturated fat and low in cholesterol and is adequate in all nutrients, including protein, carbohydrate, fat, vitamins, and minerals.

Guidelines for Lowering High Blood Cholesterol Levels
Basic Trends

Eat less high-fat food (especially those high in saturated fat).

Replace part of the saturated fat in your diet with unsaturated fat.

Eat less high-cholesterol food.

Choose foods high in complex carbohydrates (starch and fiber).

Reduce your weight, if you are overweight.

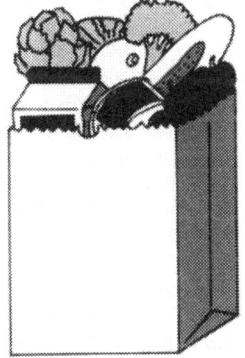

Eat Less High-Fat Food

There are two major types of dietary fat – saturated and unsaturated. Unsaturated fats are further classified as either polyunsaturated or monounsaturated fats. Together, saturated and unsaturated fats equal total fat. All foods containing fat contain a mixture of these fats.

One of the goals in your blood cholesterol-lowering diet is to eat less total fat, because this is an effective way to eat less saturated fat. Because fat is the richest source of calories, this will also help reduce the number of calories you eat every day. If you are overweight, weight loss is another important step in lowering blood cholesterol levels (as discussed later in this brochure). If you are not overweight, be sure to replace the fat calories by eating more food high in complex carbohydrates.

Remember: *When you decrease the amount of total fat you eat, you are likely to reduce the saturated fat and calories in your diet.*

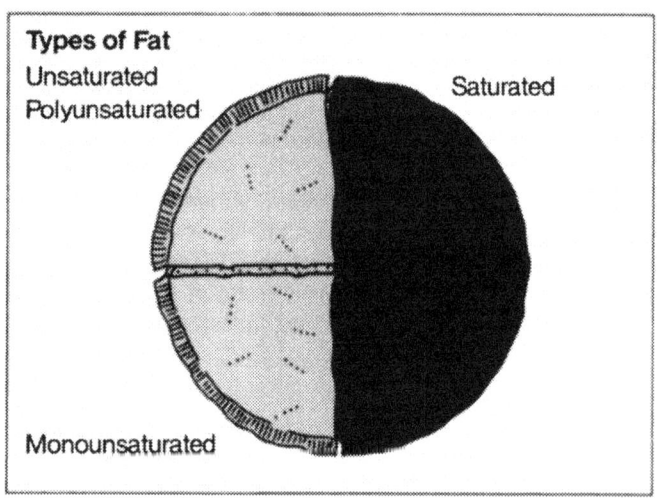

Types of Fat
Unsaturated
Polyunsaturated
Saturated
Monounsaturated

Eat Less Saturated Fat

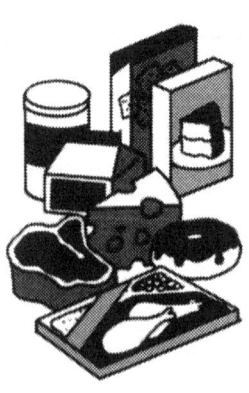

Saturated fat raises your blood cholesterol level more than anything else in your diet. The best way to reduce your blood cholesterol level is to reduce the amount of saturated fat that you eat.

Animal products as a group are a major source of saturated fat in the average American diet. Butter, cheese, whole milk, ice cream, and cream all contain high amounts of saturated fat. Saturated fat is also concentrated in the fat that surrounds meat and in the white streaks of fat in the muscle of meat (marbling). Poultry, fish, and shellfish also contain saturated fat, although generally less than meat.

A few vegetable fats – coconut oil, cocoa butter (found in chocolate), palm kernel oil, and palm oil – are high in saturated fat. These vegetable fats are found in many commercially baked goods, such as cookies and crackers, and in nondairy substitutes, such as whipped toppings, coffee creamers, cake mixes, and even frozen dinners. They also can be found in some snack foods like chips, candy bars, and buttered popcorn. Because these vegetable fats are not visible in these foods (unlike the fat in meats) it is important for you to read food labels. The label may tell you how much saturated fat a food contains, which will help you choose foods lowest in saturated fats.

Remember: *Saturated fats are found primarily in animal products. But a few vegetable fats and many commercially processed foods also contain saturated fat. Read labels carefully. Choose foods wisely.*

Substitute Unsaturated Fat for Saturated Fat

Unsaturated fat actually helps to lower cholesterol levels when it is substituted for saturated fat. Therefore, health professionals recommend that, when you do eat fats, unsaturated fats (**poly**unsaturated and **mono**unsaturated fats) be substituted for part of the saturated fat whenever possible.

Polyunsaturated fats are found primarily in safflower, corn, soybean, cottonseed, sesame, and sunflower oils, which are common cooking oils. Polyunsaturated fats are also contained in most salad dressings. But be cautious. Commercially prepared salad dressing also may be high in saturated fats, and therefore careful inspection of labels is important. The word "hydrogenated" on a label means that some of the polyunsaturated fat has been converted to saturated fat.

Another type of polyunsaturated fat is found in the oils of fish and shellfish (often referred to as fish oils, or omega-3 fatty acids). This type of polyunsaturated fat is found in greatest amounts in such fatty fish as herring, salmon, and mackerel. There is little evidence that omega-3 fatty acids are useful for reducing LDL-cholesterol levels. However, fish is a good food choice for this diet plan anyway because it is low in saturated fat. The use of fish oil supplements are not recommended for the treatment of high blood cholesterol because it is not known whether long-term ingestion of omega-3 fatty acids will lead to undesirable side effects.

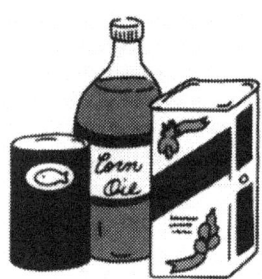

Olive and canola oil (rapeseed oil) are examples of oils that are high in **monounsaturated fats.** Like other vegetable oils, these oils are used in cooking as well as in salads. Recently, research has shown that substituting monounsaturated fat, like substituting polyunsaturated fat, for saturated fat reduces blood cholesterol levels.

Remember: *Unsaturated fats when substituted for saturated fats help lower blood cholesterol levels.*

Eat Less High-Cholesterol Food

Dietary cholesterol is a waxy, fat-like substance found in foods that come from animals. Although it is not the same as saturated fat, **dietary cholesterol also can raise your blood cholesterol level.** Therefore, it is important to eat less food that is high in cholesterol. While cholesterol is needed for normal body function, your liver makes enough for your body's needs so that you don't need to eat any cholesterol at all.

Cholesterol is found in eggs, dairy products, meat, poultry, fish, and shellfish. Egg yolks and organ meats (liver, kidney, sweetbread, brain) are particularly rich sources of cholesterol. High-fat dairy products, meat, and poultry all have similar amounts of cholesterol. Fish generally has less cholesterol, but shellfish varies in cholesterol content. Foods of plant origin, like fruits, vegetables, grains, cereals, nuts, and seeds, contain no cholesterol.

Since cholesterol is not a fat, you can find it in both high-fat and low-fat animal foods. In other words, even if a food is low in fat, it may be high in cholesterol. For instance, organ meats, like liver, are low in fat, but are high in cholesterol.

Because many foods such as dairy products and some meats are high in both saturated fat and cholesterol, it is important to limit the amount of these high-fat foods that you eat, choosing lean meats and low-fat dairy products whenever possible.

Remember: *Organ meats and egg yolks are high in cholesterol. High-fat dairy products, meat, and poultry have similar amounts of cholesterol. Some fish has less. Foods of plant origin like fruits, vegetables, vegetable oils, grains, cereals, nuts, and seeds contain no cholesterol.*

Substitute Complex Carbohydrates for Saturated Fat

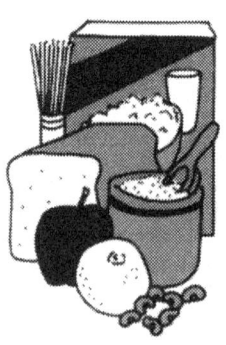

Breads, pasta, rice, cereals, dried peas and beans, fruits, and vegetables are good sources of complex carbohydrates (starch and fiber). They are excellent substitutes for foods that are high in saturated fat and cholesterol. The type of fiber found in foods such as oat and barley bran, some fruits like apples and oranges, and in some dried beans may even help reduce blood cholesterol levels.

Contrary to popular belief, **high-carbohydrate foods (like pasta, rice, potatoes) are lower in calories than foods high in fat.** In addition, they are good sources of vitamins and minerals. What adds calories to these foods is the addition of butter, rich sauces, whole milk, or cream, which are high in fat, especially saturated fat. It is important not to add these to the high-carbohydrate foods you are substituting for foods high in fat.

Remember: *Foods that are high in complex carbohydrates, if eaten plain, are low in saturated fat and cholesterol as well as being good sources of vitamins, minerals, and fiber.*

Maintain a Desirable Weight

People who are overweight frequently have higher blood cholesterol levels than people of desirable weight. You can reduce your weight by eating fewer calories and by increasing your physical activity on a regular basis. By reducing the amount of fat in your diet, you will be cutting down on the richest source of calories. Substituting foods that are high in complex carbohydrates for high-fat foods will also help you lose weight, because many high-carbohydrate foods contain little fat and thus fewer calories.

Fat has more than twice the calories as the same amount of protein or carbohydrate. Protein and carbohydrate both have about 4 calories in each gram, but all fat – saturated, polyunsaturated or monounsaturated fat – has 9 calories in each gram. **Thus, foods that are high in fat are high in calories.** And all calories count. So, to maintain a desirable weight, it is important to eat no more calories than your body needs. (To find your desirable weight, see appendix 1.)

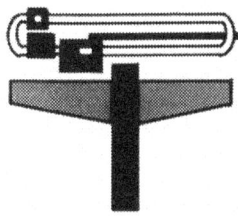

Remember: *To achieve or maintain a desirable weight, your caloric intake must not exceed the number of calories your body burns.*

How Should You Change Your Daily Menu?

So far we have discussed the basic dietary trends for reducing your blood cholesterol level. Now, we will focus on how to make specific changes in the foods you choose to eat. The following chart describes these dietary changes in terms of percentages of daily calories. (This concept is explained in the footnote.)

Since fat, carbohydrate, and protein are the three major sources of calories, the amounts that you eat of each of them makes up your daily calorie intake. For example, as shown below, the average diet of an adult American provides about 35-40 percent of calories from fat, and about 47 percent from carbohydrate and 16 percent from protein. On a cholesterol-lowering diet, the percentage of calories from total fat decreases, while the percentage of calories from carbohydrate increases and protein may stay the same.

Guidelines for Lowering Your High Blood Cholesterol Level

Specific Changes

Eat less than 30% of your total daily calories from fat.*

Less than 10% of your calories should come from saturated fat.
No more than 10% of your calories should come from polyunsaturated fat.
10-15% of your calories should come from monounsaturated fat.

Eat less than 300 mg of cholesterol each day.

Eat 50-60% of your daily calories from carbohydrates.

Adjust your caloric intake to achieve or maintain a desirable weight.

*You can calculate the percent of your total daily calories from fat with the following equations:

*You can calculate the percent of your total daily calories from fat with the following equations (use the numbers from the appendices at the end of this brochure or from food labels): % calories from fat = (total fat calories/total calories) x 100. Total fat calories = total fat (grams) x 9. In other words, if your daily calorie need is 2,000 calories, 30% of your total daily calories from fat would equal 600 calories, or 67 grams of fat.

Remember, when you are using these equations, that not **everything** you eat must have fewer than 30% calories from fat, but that you should **balance** foods with a slightly higher fat content with foods that have a much lower fat content.

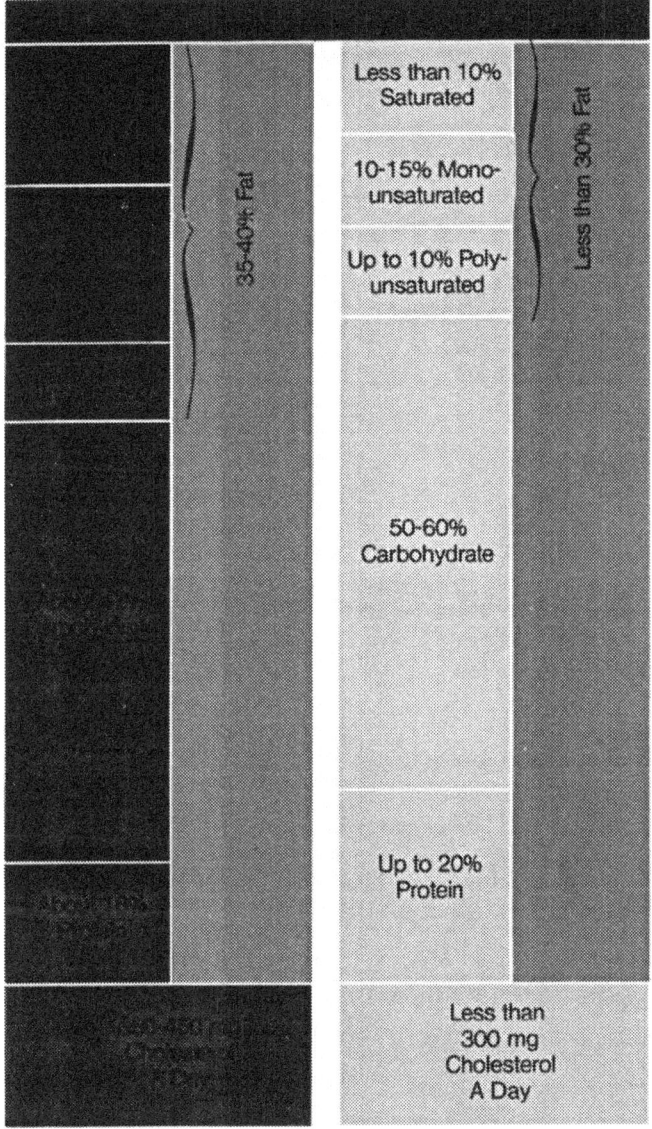

The differences between these two diets are subtle and appear to be small, but they are very important for lowering your blood cholesterol level. All of these small changes add up to big improvements in your blood cholesterol level. Take a look at the sample menus. Although the new low-fat diet has the same number of calories as the average

American diet, it has much less fat. And, the sample menus show that because the fat you were eating was so calorie-rich, the new diet actually allows you to eat more food!

Sample Menus

Average American Diet
(37% fat)

A New Low-Fat Diet
(30% fat)

Breakfast
1 fried egg
2 slices white toast
  with 1 teaspoon butter
1 cup orange juice
black coffee or tea

Breakfast
1 cup corn flakes with
  blueberries
1 cup 1% milk
1 slice rye toast
  with 1 teaspoon margarine
1 cup orange juice
black coffee or tea

Snack
1 doughnut

Snack
1 toasted pumpernickel bagel
  with 1 teaspoon margarine

Lunch
1 grilled cheese (2 ounces)
  sandwich on white bread
2 oatmeal cookies
black coffee or tea

Lunch
1 tuna salad (3 ounces) sandwich
  on whole wheat bread with
  lettuce and tomato
1 graham cracker
tea with lemon

Snack
20 cheese cracker squares

Snack
1 crisp apple

Dinner
3 ounces fried hamburger with
  ketchup
1 baked potato with sour cream
¾ cup steamed broccoli with
  1 teaspoon butter
1 cup whole milk
1 piece frosted marble cake

Dinner
3 ounces broiled lean ground
  beef with ketchup
1 baked potato with low-fat
  plain yogurt and chives
¾ cup steamed broccoli with
  1 teaspoon margarine
tossed garden salad with
  1 tablespoon oil and vinegar
  dressing
1 cup 1% milk
1 small piece homemade
  gingerbread* with a maraschino
  cherry and sprig of mint

Nutrient Analysis
Calories	2,000
Total fat (percent of calories)	37
Saturated fat (percent of calories)	19
Cholesterol	505 mg

Nutrient Analysis
Calories	2,000
Total fat (percent of calories)	30 ♥
Saturated fat (percent of calories)	10 ♥
Cholesterol	186 mg ♥

A New Low-Fat Diet
(30%)

Breakfast
1 cup shredded wheat with peach slices
1 cup 1% milk
1 slice whole wheat toast with 1 teaspoon margarine
1 cup pink grapefruit juice
black coffee

Snack
1 toasted English muffin with 1 teaspoon margarine

Lunch
3 ounces turkey salad on lettuce with tomato wedges
1 thick slice of French bread
10 animal crackers
tea with lemon

Snack
1 banana

Dinner
3 ounces broiled halibut with lemon and herb seasoning
½ cup brown rice with mushrooms
1 dinner roll with 1 teaspoon margarine
¾ cup carrot strips with 1 teaspoon margarine
spinach salad with 1 tablespoon oil and vinegar dressing
1 cup 1% milk
1 small piece homemade yellow cake*

Nutrient Analysis
Total calories	2,000
Total fat (percent of calories)	30 ♥
Saturated fat (percent of calories)	10 ♥
Cholesterol	172 mg ♥

*Homemade desserts should be made with unsaturated fats instead of saturated fats. Two egg whites may be substituted for one egg yolk.

What Kind of Success Can You Expect?

Generally your blood cholesterol level should begin to drop 2 to 3 weeks after you start on a cholesterol-lowering diet. Over time, you may reduce your level 30-55 mg/dl. The reduction in your blood cholesterol level depends on several factors:

The amount of saturated fat in your diet –
If your diet is very high in saturated fats, you will probably see a greater reduction in your cholesterol level once you start to change your eating pattern than if your initial diet was only moderately high in saturated fat.

Your blood cholesterol level prior to starting your new diet –
In general, the higher your blood cholesterol level is, the greater reduction you can expect from your new diet. If your level is very high, you might be able to lower your cholesterol level even more than 55 mg/dl.

How responsive your body is to your new diet –
Genetic factors play a role in determining your blood cholesterol level and, to some extent, can determine your ability to lower your level by diet.

How to Change Your Eating Patterns

Look at your overall eating pattern and begin to plan. If you are eating few foods high in saturated fat, an occasional high-saturated fat food won't raise your blood cholesterol level. If you anticipate a high-saturated fat, high-cholesterol day, eat an especially low-saturated fat, low-cholesterol diet the day before and the day after. With a little planning, you can change your eating patterns and reduce your high blood cholesterol level.

Remember, the goal is to limit the saturated fat and cholesterol in your diet each day. You don't have to cut out all the high-saturated fat and high-cholesterol foods in your diet. Try to substitute one or two low-saturated fat or low-cholesterol foods each day, and soon you will reach your goal of a low-saturated fat, low-cholesterol diet.

Changing your eating patterns takes time. In fact, it may take you 6 months or longer to incorporate all the changes you'll want to make in your diet. Most likely you will be shopping for some different foods, preparing some food differently, even modifying your choices at restaurants and parties.

Remember: *Eat foods high in unsaturated fats and high in complex carbohydrates in place of foods high in saturated fat and cholesterol. Make substitutions gradually and plan your meals ahead to adjust your diet and reduce your blood cholesterol level.*

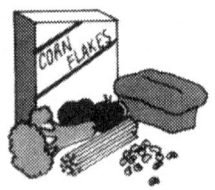

Shop for Foods That Are Low in Saturated Fat and Cholesterol

If you stock your kitchen shelves with foods that are low in saturated fat and cholesterol, it will be much easier to adjust your eating habits. With a little direction you can learn to shop for these foods.

This part of the brochure is divided into categories that will be helpful when you make out your grocery lists. The categories, or food groups, are listed in the chart below.

Food Groups

You must eat a variety of foods each day to get the nutrients you need. One way to do this is to choose foods from different food groups, which are categorized by the nutrients they provide. The number and size of portions should be adjusted to reach and maintain your desirable weight. Use the information in the following sections to identify specific foods in each of the food groups that are low in saturated fat and cholesterol.

14

Food Group

Meat, Poultry, Fish, and Shellfish
(up to 6 ounces a day)
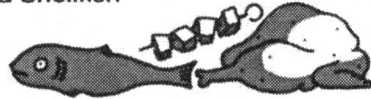

Dairy Products
(2 servings a day; 3 servings for women who are pregnant or breastfeeding)
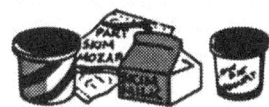

Eggs
(no more than 3 yolks a week)
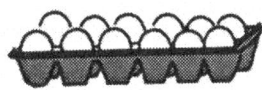

Fats and Oils
(up to 6-8 teaspoons a day)
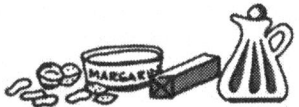

Breads, Cereals, Pasta, Rice, and Dried Peas and Beans
(6 or more servings a day)

Fruits and Vegetables
(2-4 servings of fruit, 3-5 servings of vegetables a day)
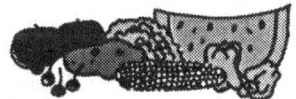

Sweets and Snacks
(avoid too many sweets)
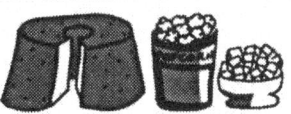

Meat, Poultry, Fish, and Shellfish

Meat, poultry, fish, and shellfish are important sources of protein and other nutrients in your diet. However, they also contain saturated fat and cholesterol. The following chart shows the differences between lean and fatty examples of each. As you can see, lean beef is lower in saturated fat than beef short ribs. Chicken without skin has less saturated fat than chicken with skin. Haddock has less saturated fat and cholesterol than either chicken or meat. And, of course, foods with less fat contain fewer calories as well.

Meat, Poultry, and Fish: A Comparison

Product (3 ounces, cooked*)	Saturated Fat (grams**)	Dietary Cholesterol (milligrams**)	Total Fat (grams**)
Beef, top round, broiled	2	84	6
Beef, short ribs, braised	8	93	18
Chicken, broiler/fryer, without skin, light meat, roasted	1	85	5
Chicken, broiler/fryer, with skin, light meat, roasted	3	85	11
Haddock, baked	0.1	63	1
Mackerel, baked	4	64	15

*About the size of a deck of cards, or ¼ pound when raw.
**The terms grams and milligrams are defined in the glossary.

To lower your blood cholesterol level, choose the leanest meats and poultry, fish, and shellfish. Remember, all of these foods contain some saturated fat and cholesterol. Therefore the amount you eat is also important. The recommended amount of meat, poultry, fish, or shellfish is up to 6 ounces each day. For variety, consider dried beans or legumes as a main dish. If larger, more filling main dishes are desired, extend meat with pasta or vegetables for hearty dishes. Eating a diet that includes a variety of foods is important because a food lowest in fat may not have the same vitamins and minerals as one a little higher in fat.

Meat. Some people think well-marbled meat (meat with white fat running through it) tastes better than less well-marbled meat. However, the tasty cuts are not all high in fat. For example, **well-trimmed cuts** from the "round" cuts of the animal are tender if prepared appropriately and they are lower in saturated fat than well-marbled meat. The list below gives you other examples of trimmed, lean meats.

Lean Cuts of Meat

Beef	Veal	Pork	Lamb
Round	All trimmed cuts except commercially ground	Tenderloin	Leg
Sirloin		Leg (fresh)	Arm
Chuck		Shoulder (arm or picnic)	Loin
Loin			

Beef, veal, and lamb can be graded as "prime," "choice," or "good." The grade is determined by the amount of marbling (fat) in the meat. "Prime," which is the top grade, has the most fat, while "choice" has less marbling. Even though the difference in marbling between "good" and "choice" is small, **"good" grades of meat are lower in fat.** Keep in mind that it is not necessary to completely remove red meat from your diet. Lean meat is high in protein and iron. Women in particular should avoid severe reductions in lean meat that would increase their risk of iron-deficiency anemia.

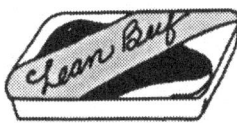

Some producers now are using "lean" and "lite" and other similar labels to designate beef, lamb, and pork that have been produced with less trimmable fat (fat surrounding the meat) and, in some instances, less marbling. These labels frequently appear on processed meat products but may appear on fresh meats as well. "Light," "lite," "leaner," and "lower fat" generally refer to foods containing less fat. They can be, but are not necessarily low in fat. Read the label for information on grams of fat per serving.

High-fat processed meats should be eaten infrequently because 60-80 percent of their calories come from fat – much of which is saturated. Some examples of these processed meats are bacon, bologna, salami, hot dogs, and sausage.

Organ meats, like liver, sweetbreads, and kidneys are relatively low in fat. However, these meats are high in cholesterol.

A more extensive list of meats is provided in appendix 2.

Poultry. In general, poultry is low in saturated fat, especially when the skin is removed. Poultry is, therefore, an excellent choice for your new diet. When choosing poultry, keep these points in mind:

- Eat chicken and turkey pieces without skin to reduce the saturated fat.
- Limit **goose, duck,** and many **processed poultry products** like bologna and hot dogs, which are very high in saturated fat.

For a more complete listing see appendix 3.

Fish and Shellfish. Most fish is lower in saturated fat and cholesterol than meat and poultry. Therefore, usually a good substitute for meats and poultry.

Shellfish varies in cholesterol content – some is relatively high and some is low – but all has less fat than meat, poultry, and most fish.

A more complete listing of seafood appears in appendix 4.

Dairy Products

Although many people believe that meats have the highest cholesterol and saturated fat content, dairy products that contain fat are also high in saturated fat and cholesterol. Since dairy products are often added to foods like casseroles, cakes, or pies, you might eat a significant amount of them without knowing it.

Milk. Milk provides many essential nutrients. And both 1% and skim milk provide the same nutrients as whole milk (3.3%) or 2% milk, while providing much less saturated fat and cholesterol and fewer calories.

Ease Your Way From Whole Milk to Skim Milk. Make the change gradually. Drink 2% milk for a few weeks, then 1%, and finally skim. With each step, you will decrease your intake of saturated fat, cholesterol, and calories.

Cheese. Often, when people cut back on meat, they replace it with cheese, thinking they are cutting back on their saturated fat and dietary cholesterol. They couldn't be more wrong. Because they are prepared from whole milk or cream, **most cheeses, while high in calcium, are also high in saturated fat and cholesterol.** Ounce for ounce, meat, poultry, and most cheeses have about the same amount of cholesterol. But cheeses for the most part have much more saturated fat. Also, cheese is not as good a source of some vitamins and minerals, especially iron, as meats. The following chart compares the saturated fat and cholesterol content in chicken, a relatively lean cut of meat, and some cheeses.

Poultry, Meat, and Cheese: A Comparison

Product (3 ounce serving)		**Saturated Fat** (grams)	**Dietary Cholesterol** (milligrams)	**Total Fat** (grams)
Beef, top round, lean only, broiled	♥	2	84	6
Chicken, broiler/fryer, without skin, light meat roasted	♥	1	85	5
Low-fat cottage cheese	♥	1	4	1
Part-skim mozzarella	♥	9	48	14
Mozzarella		11	66	18
American processed		17	81	26
Natural cheddar		18	90	28
Cream cheese		19	93	30

Determining which cheeses are high and low in saturated fat and cholesterol can be confusing because there are so many different kinds on the market: part-skim-milk, low-fat, imitation, processed, natural, hard, and soft. Imitation cheeses made with vegetable oil, part-skim-milk cheeses, and cheeses advertised as "low-fat" are usually lower in saturated fat and cholesterol than are natural and processed cheeses, which are made with whole milk. However, even part-skim-milk cheeses and "low-fat" cheeses are not necessarily lower in fat than many meats. Remember it this way:

- **Natural and processed hard cheeses** are highest in saturated fat.
- **Low-fat and imitation cheeses** may have less saturated fat.
- **Meats** have less saturated fat than many of these cheeses.

Therefore, substitute low-fat and imitation cheeses whenever possible for natural, processed, and hard cheeses. Read the label and choose low-fat cheeses that have between 2 and 6 grams of fat per ounce. When you get the urge for cheese, the following should be eaten instead of hard cheese, or low-fat imitation cheese:

Cottage cheese (low-fat)
Farmer cheese (made with skim milk)
Pot cheese

The list in appendix 5 compares the saturated fat and cholesterol content in a wide variety of dairy products.

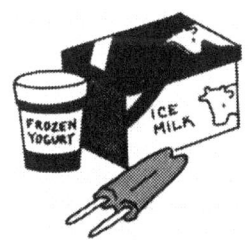

Ice Cream. Americans love ice cream. But, ice cream is made from whole milk and cream and therefore contains a considerable amount of saturated fat and dietary cholesterol. You do not need to eliminate ice cream, but do eat it in small amounts and less often. Try frozen desserts like ice milk, yogurt, sorbets, and popsicles which are low in saturated fat. Appendix 6 compares the saturated fat and cholesterol content of several frozen desserts.

Eggs

Egg **yolks** are high in cholesterol: each contains about 270 mg. Eat no more than three egg yolks a week including those in processed foods and many baked goods. Egg **whites** contain no cholesterol and can be substituted for whole eggs in recipes. For cakes or cookies, this substitution will be acceptable for 1-2 eggs in most recipes and up to 3-4 whole eggs in some.

Fats and Oils

In your cooking, limit the amounts you use of these saturated fats:

- Butter
- Lard
- Fatback
- Solid Shortenings

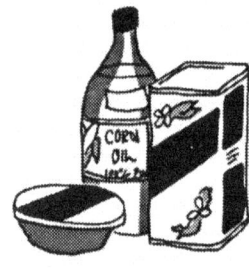

Instead of using butter as a spread or in recipes, substitute margarine. Choose liquid vegetable oils that are highest in unsaturated fats like safflower, sunflower, corn, olive, sesame, and soybean oils for your cooking and in your salad dressings. Peanut oil and peanut butter may be eaten in small amounts. Choose margarines and oils that have more polyunsaturated fat than saturated fat.

Saturated fats often are found in commercially prepared products. Remember, some vegetable oils (like coconut, palm, and palm kernel oil) are saturated, and other vegetable oils can become saturated by hydrogenation – a process that solidifies them. They are called hydrogenated vegetable oils. Read the labels before deciding which products to buy.

Appendix 7 ranks solid fats and oils from low to high in terms of saturated fat. You will reduce your intake of saturated fat by not choosing those fats at the bottom of the list. And using less will decrease your total fat intake.

Since avocados, olives, nuts, and seeds are high in fat, they are often grouped with fats and oils. Although the fat in nuts and seeds is mostly unsaturated fat, they are very high in calories. See appendix 8 to compare fat and calorie content of nuts and seeds.

Fruits and Vegetables

Fruits and vegetables contain no cholesterol and are very low in fat and low in calories (except for avocados and olives, which are high in fat and calories). By eating fruits as a snack or dessert and vegetables as snacks and side dishes, you can increase your intake of vitamins, minerals, and fiber and lower your intake of saturated fat and dietary cholesterol.

Breads, Cereals, Pasta, Rice, and Dried Peas and Beans

Breads, cereals, pasta, rice, and dried peas and beans are all high in complex carbohydrates and low in saturated fat. By substituting more foods from this group for high-saturated fat foods, you will:

- Decrease your saturated fat, dietary cholesterol, and calorie intake and
- Increase your complex carbohydrate consumption.

Try pasta, rice, and dried peas and beans (like split peas, lentils, kidney beans, and navy beans) as main dishes, casseroles, soups, or other one-dish meals without high-fat sauces. Also, try recipes that use small quantities of meat, poultry, fish, or shellfish as flavoring or seasoning in casseroles rather than as the main ingredient.

Cereal products, both cooked and dry, are usually low in saturated fat – with the exception of those that contain coconut or coconut oil, like many types of granola. (Most granolas are high in fat.)

Breads and most rolls also are low in fat (for more fiber, choose the whole-grain types). However, many other types of commercially baked goods are made with large amounts of saturated fats. Read the labels on these products to determine their fat content. The ones listed below (as well as many others) are high in saturated fat:

- Croissants
- Biscuits
- Doughnuts
- Muffins
- Butter rolls

Remember, you can make your own muffins and quick breads using unsaturated vegetable oils and egg whites. Two egg whites may be substituted for one egg yolk.

Appendix 9 lists many common foods from this group. Use it to choose those that are lowest in saturated fat and dietary cholesterol.

Sweets and Snacks   Sweets and snacks often are high in saturated fat, cholesterol, and calories. Examples of these foods are commercial cakes, pies, cookies, cheese crackers, and some types of chips. Once again, the key is to read labels carefully since some of these products may contain unsaturated fats and be low in total fat and calories.

If you are accustomed to eating commercially prepared pies, cakes, or cookies, there are some very tasty alternatives to these high-saturated fat and high-cholesterol items. A few examples of commercially prepared desserts that are acceptable include angel food cake, fig bars, and ginger snaps. Keep in mind that most desserts can be made at home substituting polyunsaturated oil or margarine for butter and lard, skim milk for whole milk, and egg whites for egg yolks (see "Low-Fat Cooking Tips"). Although this reduces their saturated fat and cholesterol content, these baked products remain a rich source of fat (and therefore calories) and should be eaten only occasionally if you are trying to lose weight. As an alternative, try fruit for dessert. And for your next snack, try a piece of fruit, some vegetables, or a low-fat snack like unbuttered popcorn or breadsticks.

See appendix 6 for more information on frozen desserts and appendix 10 for information on sweets and snacks.

Read the Labels When you are shopping, compare labels. Some premixed, frozen, or prepared foods have a lower saturated fat or cholesterol content than others. Now that many products list their fat and cholesterol content, shopping for low-saturated fat, low-cholesterol foods is much easier. With a little guidance, you can learn how to use these labels when you shop.

Look at the Ingredients All food labels list the product's ingredients in order by weight. The ingredient in the greatest amount is listed first. The ingredient in the least amount is listed last. To avoid too much total or saturated fat, limit your use of products that list a fat or oil first or that list many fat and oil ingredients. The checklist below helps you identify the names of common saturated fat and cholesterol sources in foods.

Sources of Saturated Fat and Cholesterol		
Animal Fat	Egg and Egg-Yolk Solids	Palm Kernel Oil
Bacon Fat		Palm Oil
Beef Fat	Ham Fat	Pork Fat
Butter	Hardened Fat or Oil	Turkey Fat
Chicken Fat		Vegetable Oil*
Cocoa Butter	Hydrogenated Vegetable Oil	Vegetable Shortening
Coconut		
Coconut Oil	Lamb Fat	Whole-Milk Solids
Cream	Lard	
	Meat Fat	

*Could be coconut or palm oil.

Read the Nutrition Information Look for the amount of fat, polyunsaturated, and saturated fats and cholesterol. The following samples show you how to identify products with lower saturated fat and cholesterol. The labels give the amount of fat in grams (g) and cholesterol in milligrams (mg) per serving. You can see that skim milk has less fat and cholesterol than whole milk. Tub margarine has less saturated fat and cholesterol than butter.

	Whole Milk	2% Milk	Skim Milk
Nutrition Information Per Serving			
Serving Size	1 cup	1 cup	1 cup
Calories	150	121	86
Protein	8 g	8 g	8 g
Carbohydrates	11 g	12 g	12 g
Fat	8 g	5 g	less than 1 g
Polyunsaturates	less than 1 g	less than 1 g	0 g
Saturates	5 g	3 g	less than 1 g
Cholesterol	33 mg	18 mg	4 mg

	Butter, Stick	Margarine, Tub
Nutrition Information Per Serving		
Serving Size	1 T	1 T
Calories	101	101
Protein	0.1 g	0.1 g
Carbohydrates	0.1 g	0 1 g
Fat (100% calories from fat)	11.4 g	11.4 g
Polyunsaturates	0.4 g	3.9 g
Saturates	7.1 g	1.8 g
Cholesterol	31 mg	0 mg

Note: The amount of monounsaturated fat is not listed.

Low-Fat Cooking Tips

Your kitchen is now stocked with great tasting, low-saturated fat, low-cholesterol foods. But you may still be faced with the temptation to fix your favorite higher fat meats, rich soups, and baked breads and cookies. The suggestions below will help you to reduce the amount of total and saturated fats in these foods.

New Ways To Prepare Meat, Poultry, Fish, and Shellfish

When you prepare meats, poultry, and fish, remove as much saturated fat as possible. Trim the visible fat from meat. Remove the skin and fat from the chicken, turkey, and other poultry. And, if you buy tuna or other fish that is packed in oil, rinse it in a strainer before making tuna salad or a casserole, or buy it packed in water.

Changes in your cooking style can also help you remove fat. Rather than frying meats, poultry, fish, and shellfish, try broiling, roasting, poaching, or baking. Broiling browns meats without adding fat. When you roast, place the meat on a rack so that the fat can drip away.

Finally, if you baste your roast, use fat-free ingredients such as wine, tomato juice, or lemon juice instead of the fatty drippings. If you baste turkeys and chickens with fat use vegetable oil or margarine instead of the traditional butter or lard. Self-basting turkeys can be high in saturated fat–read the label!

New Ways To Make Sauces and Soups

Sauces, including gravies and homemade pasta sauces, and many soups often can be prepared with much less fat. Before thickening a sauce or serving soup, let the stock or liquid cool – preferably in the refrigerator. The fat will rise to the top and it can easily be skimmed off. Treat canned broth-type soups the same way.

For sauces that call for sour cream, substitute plain low-fat yogurt. To prevent the yogurt from separating, mix 1 tablespoon of cornstarch with 1 tablespoon of yogurt and mix that into the rest of the yogurt. Stir over medium heat just until the yogurt thickens. Serve immediately. Also, whenever you make creamed soup or white sauces, use skim or 1% milk instead of 2% or whole milk.

New Ways To Use Old Recipes

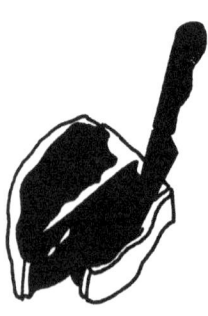

There are dozens of cookbooks and recipe booklets that will help you with low-fat cooking. But there is no reason to stop using your own favorite cookbook. The following list summarizes many of the tips. Using them, you can change tried and true recipes to low-saturated fat, low-cholesterol recipes. In some cases, especially with baked products, the quality or texture may change. For example, using vegetable oil instead of shortening in cakes that require creaming will affect the result. Use margarine instead; oil is best used only in recipes calling for **melted** butter. Substituting yogurt for sour cream sometimes affects the taste of the product. Experiment! Find the recipes that work best with these substitutions.

Instead of	**Use**
1 tablespoon butter	1 tablespoon margarine or ¾ tablespoons oil
1 cup shortening	⅔ cup vegetable oil
1 whole egg	2 egg whites
1 cup sour cream	1 cup yogurt (plus 1 tablespoon cornstarch for some recipes)
1 cup whole milk	1 cup skim milk

Where Can You Go for Help?

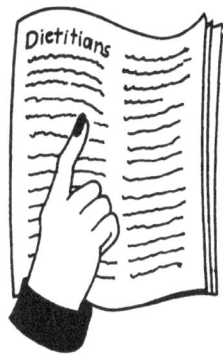

If you want additional help in planning an approach to low-saturated fat, low-cholesterol eating, make an appointment with a registered dietitian or qualified nutritionist. They can help you design an eating plan particular to your own needs and preferences. Dietitians may be identified through a local hospital as well as through state and district affiliates of the American Dietetic Association. The American Dietetic Association maintains a roster of registered dietitians. By calling the Division of Practice [(312) 899-0040] you can request names of qualified dietitians in your area. Others can be found in public health departments, health maintenance organizations, cooperative extension services, and colleges.

These health professionals can assist you in making dietary changes by providing additional advice on shopping and preparing foods, eating away from home, and changing your eating behaviors to help you maintain your new eating pattern. Their expertise will help you set short-term goals for dietary change so that you can successfully lower your high blood cholesterol levels without drastically changing your eating pattern or overall lifestyle.

If you would like more information to help you start your new approach to healthy eating, contact the National Cholesterol Education Program (NCEP) of the National Heart, Lung, and Blood Institute. NCEP has developed a *Community Guide to Cholesterol Resources,* which includes the names and addresses of other organizations that can provide additional information. *So You Have High Blood Cholesterol* provides more specific information on the significance of high blood cholesterol and how it affects your health. To request additional information, write:

National Cholesterol Education Program
National Heart, Lung, and Blood Institute
National Institutes of Health
C-200
Bethesda, MD 20892

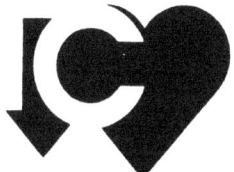

Glossary

1. **Atherosclerosis** – A type of "hardening of the arteries" in which cholesterol, fat, and other blood components build up on the inner lining of arteries. As atherosclerosis progresses, the arteries to the heart may narrow so that oxygen-rich blood and nutrients have difficulty reaching the heart.

2. **Carbohydrate** – One of the three nutrients that supply calories (energy) to the body. Carbohydrate provides 4 calories per gram—the same number of calories as pure protein and less than half the calories of fat. Carbohydrate is essential for normal body function. There are two basic kinds of carbohydrate—simple carbohydrate (or sugars) and complex carbohydrate (starches and fiber). In nature, both the simple sugars and the complex starches come packaged in foods like oranges, apples, corn, wheat, and milk. Refined or processed carbohydrates are found in cookies, cakes, and pies.

   - **Complex carbohydrate** – Starch and fiber. Complex carbohydrate comes from plants. When complex carbohydrate is substituted for saturated fat, the saturated fat reduction helps lower blood cholesterol. Foods high in starch include breads, cereals, pasta, rice, dried beans and peas, corn, and lima beans.

   - **Fiber** – A nondigestible type of complex carbohydrate. High-fiber foods are usually low in calories. Foods high in fiber include whole grain breads and cereals, whole fruits, and dried beans. The type of fiber found in foods such as oat and barley bran, some fruits like apples and oranges, and some dried beans may help reduce blood cholesterol.

3. **Cholesterol** – A soft, waxy substance. It is made in sufficient quantity by the body for normal body function, including the manufacture of hormones, bile acid, and vitamin D. It is present in all parts of the body, including the nervous system, muscle, skin, liver, intestines, heart, etc.

   - **Blood cholesterol** – Cholesterol that is manufactured in the liver and absorbed from the food you eat and is carried in the blood for use by all parts of the body. A high level of blood cholesterol leads to atherosclerosis and coronary heart disease.

- **Dietary cholesterol** – Cholesterol that is in the food you eat. It is present only in foods of animal origin, not in foods of plant origin. Dietary cholesterol, like saturated fat, tends to raise blood cholesterol, which increases the risk for heart disease.

4. **Coronary heart disease** – Heart ailment caused by narrowing of the coronary arteries (arteries that supply oxygen and nutrients directly to the heart muscle). Coronary heart disease is caused by atherosclerosis, which decreases the blood supply to the heart muscle. The inadequate supply of oxygen-rich blood and nutrients may damage the heart muscle and can lead to chest pain, heart attack, and death.

5. **Fat** – One of the three nutrients that supply calories to the body. Fat provides 9 calories per gram, more than twice the number provided by carbohydrate or protein. In addition to providing calories, fat helps in the absorption of certain vitamins. Small amounts of fat are necessary for normal body function.

    - **Total fat** – The sum of the saturated, monounsaturated, and polyunsaturated fats present in food. A mixture of all three in varying amounts is found in most foods.

    - **Saturated fat** – A type of fat found in greatest amounts in foods from animals such as meat, poultry, and whole-milk dairy products like cream, milk, ice cream, and cheese. Other examples of saturated fat include butter, the marbling and fat along the edges of meat, butter, and lard. And the saturated fat content is high in some vegetable oils—like coconut, palm kernel, and palm oils. Saturated fat raises blood cholesterol more than anything else in the diet.

    - **Unsaturated fat** – A type of fat that is usually liquid at refrigerator temperature. Monounsaturated fat and polyunsaturated fat are two kinds of unsaturated fat.

        Monounsaturated fat – A slightly unsaturated fat that is found in greatest amounts in foods from plants, including olive and canola (rapeseed) oil. When substituted for saturated fat, monounsaturated fat helps reduce blood cholesterol.

Omega-3 fatty acid (fish oil) – A type of polyunsaturated fat found in seafood and found in greatest amounts in fatty fish. Seafood is lower in saturated fat than meat.

Polyunsaturated fat – A highly unsaturated fat that is found in greatest amounts in foods from plants, including safflower, sunflower, corn, and soybean oils. When substituted for saturated fat, polyunsaturated fat helps reduce blood cholesterol.

6. **Gram (g)** – A unit of weight. There are about 28 g in 1 ounce. Dietary fat, protein, and carbohydrate are measured in grams.

7. **Hydrogenation** – A chemical process that changes liquid vegetable oils (unsaturated fat) into a more solid saturated fat. This process improves the shelf life of the product – but also increases the saturated fat content. Many commercial food products contain hydrogenated vegetable oil. Selection should be made based on information found on the label.

8. **Lipoproteins** – Protein-coated packages that carry fat and cholesterol through the blood. Lipoproteins are classified according to their density.

   - **High density lipoproteins (HDL)** – Lipoproteins that contain a small amount of cholesterol and carry cholesterol away from body cells and tissues to the liver for excretion from the body. Low levels of HDL are associated with an increased risk of coronary heart disease. Therefore the higher the HDL level, the better.

   - **Low density lipoproteins (LDL)** – Lipoproteins that contain the largest amount of cholesterol in the blood. LDL is responsible for depositing cholesterol in the artery walls. High levels of LDL are associated with an increased risk of coronary heart disease.

9. **Milligram (mg)** – A unit of weight equal to one-thousandth of a gram. There are about 28,350 mg in 1 ounce. Dietary cholesterol is measured in milligrams.

10. **Milligrams/deciliter (mg/dl)** – A way of expressing concentration: in blood cholesterol measurements, the weight of cholesterol (in milligrams) in a deciliter of blood. A deciliter is about one-tenth of a quart.

11. **Protein** – One of the three nutrients that supply calories to the body. Protein provides 4 calories per gram, which is less than half the calories of fat. Protein is an essential nutrient that becomes a component of many parts of the body, including muscle, bone, skin, and blood.

Appendix 1: Desirable Weights[1] for Men and Women (Ages 25 and Over)

	Height[2] Feet Inches		Small Frame	Medium Frame	Large Frame
Men	5	2	112-120	118-129	126-141
	5	3	115-123	121-133	129-144
	5	4	118-126	124-136	132-148
	5	5	121-129	127-139	135-152
	5	6	124-133	130-143	138-156
	5	7	128-137	134-147	142-161
	5	8	132-141	138-152	147-166
	5	9	136-145	142-156	151-170
	5	10	140-150	146-160	155-174
	5	11	144-154	150-165	159-179
	6	0	148-158	154-170	164-184
	6	1	152-162	158-175	168-189
	6	2	156-167	162-180	173-194
	6	3	160-171	167-185	178-199
	6	4	164-175	172-190	182-204
Women	4	10	92-98	96-107	104-119
	4	11	94-101	98-110	106-122
	5	0	96-104	101-113	109-125
	5	1	99-107	104-116	112-128
	5	2	102-110	107-119	115-131
	5	3	105-113	110-122	118-134
	5	4	108-116	113-126	121-138
	5	5	111-119	116-130	125-142
	5	6	114-123	120-135	129-146
	5	7	118-127	124-139	133-150
	5	8	122-131	128-143	137-154
	5	9	126-135	132-147	141-158
	5	10	130-140	136-151	145-163
	5	11	134-144	140-155	149-168
	6	0	138-148	144-159	153-173

[1] Weight in pounds according to frame (indoor clothing).
[2] With 1-inch heel shoes on for men and 2-inch heel shoes on for women.

SOURCE: Metropolitan Life Insurance Company Actuarial Tables, 1959.

Appendix 2: Meats
Fat and Cholesterol Comparison Chart

When following a cholesterol-lowering diet, select the meats that are lowest in saturated fat (i.e. saturated fatty acids) and cholesterol. The information on total fat, percent calories from fat, and calories should be helpful if you are trying to lose weight.

The following foods within each category (veal, lamb, beef, pork) are ranked from low to high saturated fat. To reduce the saturated fat in your diet, select the leaner cuts from the upper portion of each category. Trimming the visible fat will reduce the fat content even more. Since meats contribute a significant amount of saturated fat and cholesterol to your diet, you should eat smaller portions (no more than 6 ounces a day).

Product (3½ Ounces, Cooked)*	Saturated Fatty Acids (Grams)	Cholesterol (Milligrams)	Total Fat[1] (Grams)	Calories From Fat[2] (%)	Total Calories
Beef					
Kidneys, simmered[3]	1.1	387	3.4	21	144
Liver, braised[3]	1.9	389	4.9	27	161
Round, top round, lean only, broiled	2.2	84	6.2	29	191
Round, eye of round, lean only, roasted	2.5	69	6.5	32	183
Round, tip round, lean only, roasted	2.8	81	7.5	36	190
Round, full cut, lean only, choice, broiled	2.9	82	8.0	37	194
Round, bottom round, lean only, braised	3.4	96	9.7	39	222
Short loin, top loin, lean only, broiled	3.6	76	8.9	40	203
Wedge-bone sirloin, lean only, broiled	3.6	89	8.7	38	208
Short loin, tenderloin, lean only, broiled	3.6	84	9.3	41	204
Chuck, arm pot roast, lean only, braised	3.8	101	10.0	39	231

Product (3½ Ounces, Cooked)*	Saturated Fatty Acids (Grams)	Cholesterol (Milligrams)	Total Fat[1] (Grams)	Calories From Fat[2] (%)	Total Calories
Short loin, T-bone steak, lean only, choice, broiled	4.2	80	10.4	44	214
Short loin, porterhouse steak, lean only, choice, broiled	4.3	80	10.8	45	218
Brisket, whole, lean only, braised	4.6	93	12.8	48	241
Rib eye, small end (ribs 10-12), lean only, choice, broiled	4.9	80	11.6	47	225
Rib, whole (ribs 6-12), lean only, roasted	5.8	81	13.8	52	240
Flank, lean only, choice, braised	5.9	71	13.8	51	244
Rib, large end (ribs 6-9), lean only, broiled	6.1	82	14.2	55	233
Chuck, blade roast, lean only, braised	6.2	106	15.3	51	270
Corned beef, cured, brisket, cooked	6.3	98	19.0	68	251
Flank, lean and fat, choice, braised	6.6	72	15.5	54	257
Ground, lean, broiled medium	7.2	87	18.5	61	272
Round, full cut, lean and fat, choice, braised	7.3	84	18.2	60	274
Rib, short ribs, lean only, choice, braised	7.7	93	18.1	55	295
Salami, cured, cooked, smoked, 3-4 slices	9.0	65	20.7	71	262
Short loin, T-bone steak, lean and fat, choice, broiled	10.2	84	24.6	68	324

Product (3½ Ounces, Cooked)*	Saturated Fatty Acids (Grams)	Cholesterol (Milligrams)	Total Fat[1] (Grams)	Calories From Fat[2] (%)	Total Calories
Chuck, arm pot roast, lean and fat, braised	10.7	99	26.0	67	350
Sausage, cured, cooked, smoked, about 2	11.4	67	26.9	78	312
Bologna, cured, 3-4 slices	12.1	58	28.5	82	312
Frankfurter, cured, about 2	12.0	61	28.5	82	315
Lamb					
Leg, lean only, roasted	3.0	89	8.2	39	191
Loin chop, lean only, broiled	4.1	94	9.4	39	215
Rib, lean only, roasted	5.7	88	12.3	48	232
Arm chop, lean only, braised	6.0	122	14.6	47	279
Rib, lean and fat, roasted	14.2	90	30.6	75	368
Pork					
Cured, ham steak, boneless, extra lean, unheated	1.4	45	4.2	31	122
Liver, braised[3]	1.4	355	4.4	24	165
Kidneys, braised[3]	1.5	480	4.7	28	151
Fresh, loin, tenderloin, lean only, roasted	1.7	93	4.8	26	166
Cured, shoulder, arm picnic, lean only, roasted	2.4	48	7.0	37	170
Cured, ham, boneless, regular, roasted	3.1	59	9.0	46	178
Fresh, leg (ham), shank half, lean only, roasted	3.6	92	10.5	44	215

Product (3½ Ounces, Cooked)*	Saturated Fatty Acids (Grams)	Cholesterol (Milligrams)	Total Fat[1] (Grams)	Calories From Fat[2] (%)	Total Calories
Fresh, leg (ham), rump half, lean only, roasted	3.7	96	10.7	43	221
Fresh, loin, center loin, sirloin, lean only, roasted	4.5	91	13.1	49	240
Fresh, loin, sirloin, lean only, roasted	4.5	90	13.2	50	236
Fresh, loin, center rib, lean only, roasted	4.8	79	13.8	51	245
Fresh, loin, top loin, lean only, roasted	4.8	79	13.8	51	245
Fresh, shoulder, blade, Boston, lean only, roasted	5.8	98	16.8	59	256
Fresh, loin, blade, lean only, roasted	6.6	89	19.3	62	279
Fresh, loin, sirloin, lean and fat, roasted	7.4	91	20.4	63	291
Cured, shoulder, arm picnic, lean and fat, roasted	7.7	58	21.4	69	280
Fresh, loin, center loin, lean and fat, roasted	7.9	91	21.8	64	305
Cured, shoulder, blade roll, lean and fat, roasted	8.4	67	23.5	74	287
Fresh, Italian sausage, cooked	9.0	78	25.7	72	323
Fresh, bratwurst, cooked	9.3	60	25.9	77	301
Fresh, chitterlings, cooked	10.1	143	28.8	86	303
Cured, liver sausage, liverwurst	10.6	158	28.5	79	326
Cured, smoked link sausage, grilled	11.3	68	31.8	74	389

Product (3½ Ounces, Cooked)*	Saturated Fatty Acids (Grams)	Cholesterol (Milligrams)	Total Fat[1] (Grams)	Calories From Fat[2] (%)	Total Calories
Fresh, spareribs, lean and fat, braised	11.8	121	30.3	69	397
Cured, salami, dry or hard	11.9	—	33.7	75	407
Bacon, fried	17.4	85	49.2	78	576
Veal					
Rump, lean only, roasted	—	128	2.2	13	156
Sirloin, lean only, roasted	—	128	3.2	19	153
Arm steak, lean only, cooked	—	90	5.3	24	200
Loin chop, lean only, cooked	—	90	6.7	29	207
Blade, lean only, cooked	—	90	7.8	33	211
Cutlet, medium fat, braised or broiled	4.8	128	11.0	37	271
Foreshank, medium fat, stewed	—	90	10.4	43	216
Plate, medium fat, stewed	—	90	21.2	63	303
Rib, medium fat, roasted	7.1	128	16.9	70	218
Flank, medium fat, stewed	—	90	32.3	75	390

*3½ ozs = 100 grams (approximately)

[1]Total fat = saturated fatty acids plus monounsaturated fatty acids plus polyunsaturated fatty acids.

[2]Percent calories from fat = (total fat calories divided by total calories) multiplied by 100; total fat calories = total fat (grams) multiplied by 9.

[3]Liver and most organ meats are low in fat, but high in cholesterol. If you are eating to lower your blood cholesterol, you should consider your total cholesterol intake before selecting an organ meat.

— = Information not available in the sources used.

Sources:
Composition of Foods: Beef Products – Raw • Processed • Prepared, Agriculture Handbook 8-13. United States Department of Agriculture, Human Nutrition Information Service (August 1986).

Composition of Foods: Pork Products – Raw • Processed • Prepared, Agriculture Handbook 8-10. United States Department of Agriculture, Human Nutrition Information Service (August 1983).

Home and Garden Bulletin. Nutritive Value of Foods. No. 72. United States Department of Agriculture. Human Nutrition Information Service (1986).

Appendix 3: Poultry Fat and Cholesterol Comparison Chart

When following a cholesterol-lowering diet, select poultry low in saturated fat (i.e. saturated fatty acids) and cholesterol. Choosing poultry lower in total fat, calories, and percent calories from fat will also help you lose weight.

This table ranks poultry from low to high saturated fat. Select the lower fat poultry from the upper portion of the table. In general, poultry, especially poultry with the skin removed, is lower in saturated fat than most cuts of meat. To reduce the saturated fat in your diet even more, eat smaller servings (no more than 6 ounces a day).

Product (3½ Ounces, Cooked)*	Saturated Fatty Acids (Grams)	Cholesterol (Milligrams)	Total Fat[1] (Grams)	Calories From Fat[2] (%)	Total Calories
Turkey, fryer-roasters, light meat without skin, roasted	0.4	86	1.9	8	140
Chicken, roasters, light meat without skin, roasted	1.1	75	4.1	24	153
Turkey, fryer-roasters, light meat with skin, roasted	1.3	95	4.6	25	164
Chicken, broilers or fryers, light meat without skin, roasted	1.3	85	4.5	24	173
Turkey, fryer-roasters, dark meat without skin, roasted	1.4	112	4.3	24	162
Chicken, stewing, light meat without skin, stewed	2.0	70	8.0	34	213
Turkey roll, light and dark	2.0	55	7.0	42	149

Product (3½ Ounces, Cooked)*	Saturated Fatty Acids (Grams)	Cholesterol (Milligrams)	Total Fat[1] (Grams)	Calories From Fat[2] (%)	Total Calories
Turkey, fryer-roasters, dark meat with skin, roasted	2.1	117	7.1	35	182
Chicken, roasters, dark meat without skin, roasted	2.4	75	8.8	44	178
Chicken, broilers or fryers, dark meat without skin, roasted	2.7	93	9.7	43	205
Chicken, broilers or fryers, light meat with skin, roasted	3.0	85	10.9	44	222
Chicken, stewing, dark meat without skin, stewed	4.1	95	15.3	53	258
Duck, domesticated, flesh only, roasted	4.2	89	11.2	50	201
Chicken, broilers or fryers, dark meat with skin, roasted	4.4	91	15.8	56	253
Goose, domesticated, flesh only, roasted	4.6	96	12.7	48	238
Turkey bologna, about 3½ slices	5.1	99	15.2	69	199
Chicken frankfurter, about 2	5.5	101	19.5	68	257
Turkey frankfurter, about 2	5.9	107	17.7	70	226

*3½ ozs = 100 grams (approximately)
[1]Total fat = saturated fatty acids plus monounsaturated fatty acids plus polyunsaturated fatty acids.
[2]Percent calories from fat = (total fat calories divided by total calories) multiplied by 100; total fat calories = total fat (grams) multiplied by 9.
Source:
Composition of Foods: Poultry Products – Raw • Processed • Prepared, Agriculture Handbook 8-5. United States Department of Agriculture, Science and Education Administration (August 1979).

Appendix 4: Fish and Shellfish Fat and Cholesterol Comparison Chart

When following a cholesterol-lowering diet, you may want to eat more fish and shellfish, which in general have a lot less saturated fat (i.e. saturated fatty acids) and cholesterol than meat and poultry. However, some shellfish is relatively high in cholesterol and should be eaten less often. Fish and shellfish also contain less total fat and calories than meat and poultry. Use the information on total fat, percent calories from fat, and calories to help you lose weight.

This table ranks fish and shellfish within each category (finfish, crustaceans, mollusks) from low to high saturated fat. You will want to select the lower fat and cholesterol fish and shellfish from the upper portion of the table. To reduce the amount of saturated fat in your diet even more, eat smaller portions (no more than 6 ounces a day).

Omega-3 fatty acid (fish oil) is a type of polyunsaturated fat found in the greatest amounts in fattier fish. Evidence is mounting that omega-3 fatty acids in the diet may help lower high blood cholesterol. Since their potential benefit is not fully understood, the use of fish oil supplements is not recommended. However, eating fish is beneficial because it not only contains omega-3 fatty acids but, more importantly, it is low in saturated fat.

Product (3½ Ounces Cooked)*	Saturated Fatty Acids (Grams)	Cholesterol (Milligrams)	Omega-3 Fatty Acids (Grams)	Total Fat[1] (Grams)	Calories From Fat[2] (%)	Total Calories
Finfish						
Haddock, dry heat	0.2	74	0.2	0.9	7	112
Cod, Atlantic, dry heat	0.2	55	0.2	0.9	7	105
Pollock, walleye, dry heat	0.2	96	1.5	1.1	9	113
Perch, mixed species, dry heat	0.2	42	0.3	1.2	9	117
Grouper, mixed species, dry heat	0.3	47	—	1.3	10	118
Whiting, mixed species, dry heat	0.3	84	0.9	1.7	13	115
Snapper, mixed species, dry heat	0.4	47	—	1.7	12	128
Halibut, Atlantic and Pacific, dry heat	0.4	41	0.6	2.9	19	140

Product (3½ Ounces Cooked)*	Saturated Fatty Acids (Grams)	Cholesterol (Milligrams)	Omega-3 Fatty Acids (Grams)	Total Fat[1] (Grams)	Calories From Fat[2] (%)	Total Calories
Rockfish, Pacific, dry heat	0.5	44	0.5	2.0	15	121
Sea bass, mixed species, dry heat	0.7	53	—	2.5	19	124
Trout, rainbow, dry heat	0.8	73	0.9	4.3	26	151
Swordfish, dry heat	1.4	50	1.1	5.1	30	155
Tuna, bluefin, dry heat	1.6	49	—	6.3	31	184
Salmon, sockeye, dry heat	1.9	87	1.3	11.0	46	216
Anchovy, European, canned	2.2	—	2.1	9.7	42	210
Herring, Atlantic, dry heat	2.6	77	2.1	11.5	51	203
Eel, dry heat	3.0	161	0.7	15.0	57	236
Mackerel, Atlantic, dry heat	4.2	75	1.3	17.8	61	262
Pompano, Florida, dry heat	4.5	64	—	12.1	52	211
Crustaceans						
Lobster, northern	0.1	72	0.1	0.6	6	98
Crab, blue, moist heat	0.2	100	0.5	1.8	16	102
Shrimp, mixed species, moist heat	0.3	195	0.3	1.1	10	99
Mollusks						
Whelk, moist heat	0.1	130	—	0.8	3	275
Clam, mixed species, moist heat	0.2	67	0.3	2.0	12	148
Mussel, blue, moist heat	0.9	56	0.8	4.5	23	172
Oyster, Eastern, moist heat	1.3	109	1.0	5.0	33	137

*3½ ozs = 100 grams (approximately).
[1]Total fat = saturated fatty acids plus monounsaturated fatty acids plus polyunsaturated fatty acids.
[2]Percent calories from fat = (total fat calories divided by total calories) multiplied by 100; total fat calories = total fat (grams) multiplied by 9.
— = Information not available in sources used.

Source:
Composition of Foods: Finfish and Shellfish Products--Raw • Processed • Prepared, Agriculture Handbook 8-15. United States Department of Agriculture (in press).

Appendix 5: Dairy and Egg Products Fat and Cholesterol Comparison Chart

When following a cholesterol-lowering diet, select dairy products low in saturated fat (i.e. saturated fatty acids) and cholesterol. Whole milk dairy products are relatively high in both when compared ounce for ounce with meat, poultry, and seafood. If you are trying to lose weight on your cholesterol-lowering diet, choose dairy products low in total fat, calories, and percent calories from fat.

The following foods within each category (milk, yogurt, cheese) are ranked from low to high saturated fat. In general, the hard cheeses are much higher in saturated fat and cholesterol than yogurt and most soft cheeses. You will want to select foods from the upper portion of each category.

Product	Saturated Fat (Grams)	Cholesterol (Milligrams)	Total Fat[1] (Grams)	Calories from Fat[2](%)	Total Calories
Milk (8 ounces)					
Skim milk	0.3	4	0.4	5	86
Buttermilk	1.3	9	2.2	20	99
Low-fat milk, 1% fat	1.6	10	2.6	23	102
Low-fat milk, 2% fat	2.9	18	4.7	35	121
Whole milk, 3.3% fat	5.1	33	8.2	49	150
Yogurt (4 ounces)					
Plain yogurt, low fat	0.1	2	0.2	3	63
Plain yogurt	2.4	14	3.7	47	70
Cheese					
Cottage cheese, low-fat, 1% fat, 4 oz.	0.7	5	1.2	13	82
Mozzarella, part-skim, 1 oz.	2.9	16	4.5	56	72
Cottage cheese, creamed, 4 oz.	3.2	17	5.1	39	117
Mozzarella, 1 oz.	3.7	22	6.1	69	80
Sour cream, 1 oz.	3.7	12	5.9	87	61
American processed cheese spread, pasteurized, 1 oz.	3.8	16	6.0	66	82
Feta, 1 oz.	4.2	25	6.0	72	75
Neufchatel, 1 oz.	4.2	22	6.6	81	74

Product	Saturated Fat (Grams)	Cholesterol (Milligrams)	Total Fat[1] (Grams)	Calories from Fat[2](%)	Total Calories
Camembert, 1 oz.	4.3	20	6.9	73	85
American processed cheese food, pasteurized, 1 oz.	4.4	18	7.0	68	93
Provolone, 1 oz.	4.8	20	7.6	68	100
Limburger, 1 oz.	4.8	26	7.7	75	93
Brie, 1 oz.	4.9	28	7.9	74	95
Romano, 1 oz.	4.9	29	7.6	63	110
Gouda, 1 oz.	5.0	32	7.8	69	101
Swiss, 1 oz.	5.0	26	7.8	65	107
Edam, 1 oz.	5.0	25	7.9	70	101
Brick, 1 oz.	5.3	27	8.4	72	105
Blue, 1 oz.	5.3	21	8.2	73	100
Gruyere, 1 oz.	5.4	31	9.2	71	117
Muenster, 1 oz.	5.4	27	8.5	74	104
Parmesan, 1 oz.	5.4	22	8.5	59	129
Monterey Jack, 1 oz.	5.5	25	8.6	73	106
Roquefort, 1 oz.	5.5	26	8.7	75	105
Ricotta, part-skim, 4 oz.	5.6	25	9.0	52	156
American processed cheese, pasteurized, 1 oz.	5.6	27	8.9	75	106
Colby, 1 oz.	5.7	27	9.1	73	112
Cheddar, 1 oz.	6.0	30	9.4	74	114
Cream cheese, 1 oz.	6.2	31	9.9	90	99
Ricotta, whole milk, 4 oz.	9.4	58	14.7	67	197
Eggs					
Egg, chicken, white	0	0	tr.	0	16
Egg, chicken, whole	1.7	274	5.6	64	79
Egg, chicken, yolk	1.7	272	5.6	80	63

[1]Total fat = saturated fatty acids plus monounsaturated fatty acids plus polyunsaturated fatty acids.

[2]Percent calories from fat = (total fat calories divided by total calories) multiplied by 100; total fat calories = total fat (grams) multiplied by 9.

oz. = ounce
tr. = trace

Source:
Composition of Foods: Dairy and Egg Products – Raw • Processed • Prepared, Agriculture Handbook 8-1, United States Department of Agriculture, Agricultural Research Service (November 1976).

Appendix 6: Frozen Desserts Fat and Cholesterol Comparison Chart

When following a cholesterol-lowering diet, select frozen desserts low in saturated fat (i.e. saturated fatty acids) and cholesterol. This table ranks frozen desserts from low to high saturated fat. Select the lower fat desserts from the upper portion of the list. If you are also trying to lose weight on your cholesterol-lowering diet, the calories will be of special interest to you. Although some frozen desserts are lower in fat than others, they may be just as high in calories as the higher fat products because of their sugar content. You will want to select those desserts not only low in fat but also low in calories.

Product (1 cup)	Saturated Fatty Acids (Grams)	Cholesterol (Milligrams)	Total Fat[1] (Grams)	Calories from Fat[2] (%)	Total Calories
Fruit popsicle, 1 bar	—	—	0.0	0	65
Fruit ice	—	—	tr.	0	247
Fudgsicle	—	—	0.2	2	91
Frozen yogurt, fruit flavored	—	—	2.0	8	216
Sherbet, orange	2.4	14	3.8	13	270
Pudding pops, 1 pop	2.5	1	2.6	25	94
Ice milk, vanilla, soft serve	2.9	13	4.6	19	223
Ice milk, vanilla, hard	3.5	18	5.6	28	184
Ice cream, vanilla, regular	8.9	59	14.3	48	269
Ice cream, french vanilla, soft serve	13.5	153	22.5	54	377
Ice cream, vanilla, rich, 16% fat	14.7	88	23.7	61	349

[1] Total fat = saturated fatty acids plus monounsaturated fatty acids plus polyunsaturated fatty acids.

[2] Percent calories from fat = (total fat calories divided by total calories) multiplied by 100; total fat calories = total fat (grams) multiplied by 9.

— = Information not available in sources used.

tr. = trace

Sources:
Composition of Foods: Dairy and Egg Products – Raw • Processed • Prepared, Agriculture Handbook 8-1. United States Department of Agriculture, Agricultural Research Service (November 1976).
Pennington, J., and Church, H. *Bowes and Church's Food Values of Portions Commonly Used.* 14th ed. Philadelphia: J.B. Lippincott Company (1985).

Appendix 7: Fats and Oils Comparison Chart

This table compares the fat content of selected fats and oils, going from those with a low saturated fat (i.e. saturated fatty acids) content to those with a high saturated fat content. When following a cholesterol-lowering diet, you will limit the amount of fat and oil in your diet and when necessary use those fats which are lower in saturated fat, in the upper portion of the table. All fats and oils are high in calories, 115-120 calories per tablespoon.

Product (1 Tablespoon)	Saturated Fatty Acids (Grams)	Cholesterol (Milligrams)	Polyunsaturated Fatty Acids (Grams)	Monounsaturated Fatty Acids (Grams)
Rapeseed oil (canola oil)	0.9	0	4.5	7.6
Safflower oil	1.2	0	10.1	1.6
Sunflower oil	1.4	0	5.5	6.2
Peanut butter, smooth	1.5	0	2.3	3.7
Corn oil	1.7	0	8.0	3.3
Olive oil	1.8	0	1.1	9.9
Hydrogenated sunflower oil	1.8	0	4.9	6.3
Margarine, liquid, bottled	1.8	0	5.1	3.9
Margarine, soft, tub	1.8	0	3.9	4.8
Sesame oil	1.9	0	5.7	5.4
Soybean oil	2.0	0	7.9	3.2
Margarine, stick	2.1	0	3.6	5.1
Peanut oil	2.3	0	4.3	6.2
Cottonseed oil	3.5	0	7.1	2.4
Lard	5.0	12	1.4	5.8
Beef tallow	6.4	14	0.5	5.3
Palm oil	6.7	0	1.3	5.0
Butter	7.1	31	0.4	3.3
Cocoa butter	8.1	0	0.4	4.5
Palm kernel oil	11.1	0	0.2	1.5
Coconut oil	11.8	0	0.2	0.8

Sources:

Composition of Foods: Fats and Oils – Raw • Processed • Prepared, Agriculture Handbook 8-4. United States Department of Agriculture, Science and Education Administration (June 1979).

Composition of Foods: Legumes and Legume Products – Raw • Processed • Prepared, Agriculture Handbook 8-16. United States Department of Agriculture, Human Nutrition Information Service (December 1986).

Appendix 8: Nuts and Seeds Fat Comparison Chart

When following a cholesterol-lowering diet, you will be selecting foods low in saturated fat (i.e. saturated fatty acids) and cholesterol. This table ranks nuts and seeds from low to high saturated fat. Choose those from the upper portion of the list. Most nuts and seeds would appear to be appropriate foods to eat because they contain little saturated fat. However, except for chestnuts, they are all high in total fat and consequently high in calories. Thus if you are also trying to lose weight, you should limit the use of nuts and seeds in your diet.

Product (1 ounce)	Saturated Fatty Acids (Grams)	Cholesterol (Milligrams)	Total Fat[1] (Grams)	Calories from Fat[2] (%)	Total Calories
European chestnuts	0.2	0	1.1	9	105
Filberts or hazelnuts	1.3	0	17.8	89	179
Almonds	1.4	0	15.0	80	167
Pecans	1.5	0	18.4	89	187
Sunflower seed kernels, roasted	1.5	0	1.4	77	165
English walnuts	1.6	0	17.6	87	182
Pistachio nuts	1.7	0	13.7	75	164
Peanuts	1.9	0	14.0	76	164
Hickory nuts	2.0	0	18.3	88	187
Pine nuts, pignolia	2.2	0	14.4	89	146
Pumpkin and squash seed kernels	2.3	0	12.0	73	148
Cashew nuts	2.6	0	13.2	73	163
Macadamia nuts	3.1	0	20.9	95	199
Brazil nuts	4.6	0	18.8	91	186
Coconut meat, unsweetened	16.3	0	18.3	88	187

[1]Total fat = saturated fatty acids plus monounsaturated fatty acids plus polyunsaturated fatty acids.

[2]Percent calories from fat = (total fat calories divided by total calories) multiplied by 100; total fat calories = total fat (grams) multiplied by 9.

Sources:
Composition of Foods: Legumes and Legume Products – Raw • Processed • Prepared, Agriculture Handbook 8-16. United States Department of Agriculture, Human Nutrition Information Service (December 1986).

Composition of Foods: Nut and Seed Products – Raw • Processed • Prepared, Agriculture Handbook 8-12. United States Department of Agriculture, Human Nutrition Information Service (September 1984).

Appendix 9: Breads, Cereals, Pasta, Rice, and Dried Peas and Beans Fat and Cholesterol Comparison Chart

When following a cholesterol-lowering diet, you will be selecting foods low in saturated fat (i.e. saturated fatty acids) and cholesterol. To lose weight on your cholesterol-lowering diet, choose foods that are lower in total fat, percent calories from fat, and calories.

Each of the following categories (breads, cereals, pasta, rice, and dried peas and beans) is ranked from low to high saturated fat. To reduce the saturated fat in your diet, select the products from the upper portion of each category.

Product	Saturated Fatty Acids (Grams)	Cholesterol (Milligrams)	Total Fat[1] (Grams)	Calories from Fat[2] (%)	Total Calories
Breads					
Melba toast, 1 plain	0.1	0	tr.	0	20
Pita, ½ large shell	0.1	0	1.0	5	165
Corn tortilla	0.1	0	1.0	14	65
Rye bread, 1 slice	0.2	0	1.0	14	65
English muffin	0.3	0	1.0	6	140
Bagel, 1, 3½" diameter	0.3	0	2.0	9	200
White bread, 1 slice	0.3	0	1.0	14	65
Rye krisp, 2 triple crackers	0.3	0	1.0	16	56
Whole wheat bread, 1 slice	0.4	0	1.0	13	70
Saltines, 4	0.5	4	1.0	18	50
Hamburger bun	0.5	tr.	2.0	16	115
Hot dog bun	0.5	tr.	2.0	16	115
Pancake, 1, 4" diameter	0.5	16	2.0	30	60
Bran muffin, 1, 2½" diameter	1.4	24	6.0	43	125
Corn muffin, 1, 2½" diameter	1.5	23	5.0	31	145
Plain doughnut, 1, 3¼" diameter	2.8	20	12.0	51	210
Croissant, 1, 4½" by 4"	3.5	13	12.0	46	235
Waffle, 1, 7" diameter	4.0	102	13.0	48	245

Product	Saturated Fatty Acids (Grams)	Cholesterol (Milligrams)	Total Fat[1] (Grams)	Calories from Fat[2] (%)	Total Calories
Cereals (1 cup)					
Corn flakes	tr.	—	0.1	0	98
Cream of wheat, cooked	tr.	—	0.5	3	134
Corn grits, cooked	tr.	—	0.5	3	146
Oatmeal, cooked	0.4	—	2.4	15	145
Granola	5.8	—	33.1	50	595
100% Natural Cereal with raisins and dates	13.7	—	20.3	37	496
Pasta (1 cup)					
Spaghetti, cooked	0.1	0	1.0	6	155
Elbow macaroni, cooked	0.1	0	1.0	6	155
Egg noodles, cooked	0.5	50	2.0	11	160
Chow mein noodles, canned	2.1	5	11.0	45	220
Rice (1 cup cooked)					
Rice, white	0.1	0	0.5	2	225
Rice, brown	0.3	0	1.0	4	230
Dried Peas and Beans (1 cup cooked)					
Split peas	0.1	0	0.8	3	231
Kidney beans	0.1	0	1.0	4	225
Lima beans	0.2	0	0.7	3	217
Black eyed peas	0.3	0	1.2	5	200
Garbanzo beans	0.4	0	4.3	14	269

[1]Total fat = saturated fatty acids plus monounsaturated fatty acids plus polyunsaturated fatty acids.

[2]Percent calories from fat = (total fat calories divided by total calories) multiplied by 100; total fat calories = total fat (grams) multiplied by 9.

— = Information not available in sources used.

oz. = ounce

tr. = trace

Sources:
Composition of Foods: Breakfast Cereals – Raw • Processed • Prepared, Agriculture Handbook 8-8. United States Department of Agriculture, Human Nutrition Information Service (July 1982).

Composition of Foods: Legume and Legume Products, Agriculture Handbook 8-16. United States Department of Agriculture, Nutrition Monitoring Division (December 1986).

Home and Garden Bulletin. Nutritive Value of Foods. No. 72. United States Department of Agriculture. Human Nutrition Information Service (1986).

Appendix 10: Sweets and Snacks Fat and Cholesterol Comparison Chart

When following a cholesterol-lowering diet, select foods low in saturated fat (i.e. saturated fatty acids) and cholesterol. To lose weight on your cholesterol-lowering diet, see the information on total fat, percent of calories from fat, and calories. Since the foods in this table may be sweet even if they are low in fat, they could be high in calories. Fruits, vegetables, and breads provide tasty, low-fat, low-calorie alternatives.

The following foods within each category (beverages, candy, cookies, cakes and pies, snacks, and pudding) are ranked from low to high saturated fat. To reduce the saturated fat in your diet, select the products from the upper portion of each category.

Product	Saturated Fatty Acids (Grams)	Cholesterol (Milligrams)	Total Fat[1] (Grams)	Calories from Fat[2] (%)	Total Calories
Beverages					
Ginger ale, 12 oz.	0.0	0	0.0	0	125
Cola, regular, 12 oz.	0.0	0	0.0	0	160
Chocolate shake, 10 oz.	6.5	37	10.5	26	360
Candy (1 ounce)					
Hard candy	0.0	0	0.0	0	110
Gum drops	tr.	0	tr.	tr.	100
Fudge	2.1	1	3.0	24	115
Milk chocolate, plain	5.4	6	9.0	56	145
Cookies					
Vanilla wafers, 5 cookies, 1¾" diameter	0.9	12	3.3	32	94
Fig bars, 4 cookies 1⅝" × 1⅝" × ⅜"	1.0	27	4.0	17	210
Chocolate brownie with icing, 1½" by 1¾" by ⅞"	1.6	14	4.0	36	100
Oatmeal cookies, 4 cookies, 2⅝" diameter	2.5	2	10.0	37	245
Chocolate chip cookies, 4 cookies, 2¼" diameter	3.9	18	11.0	54	185

Product	Saturated Fatty Acids (Grams)	Cholesterol (Milligrams)	Total Fat[1] (Grams)	Calories from Fat[2] (%)	Total Calories
Cakes and Pies					
Angel food cake, 1/12 of 10" cake	tr.	0	tr.	tr.	125
Gingerbread, 1/9 of 8" cake	1.1	1	4.0	21	175
White layer cake with white icing, 1/16 of 9" cake	2.1	3	9.0	32	260
Yellow layer cake with chocolate icing, 1/16 of 9" cake	3.0	36	8.0	31	235
Pound cake, 1/17 of loaf	3.0	64	5.0	41	110
Devils food cake with chocolate icing, 1/16 of 9" cake	3.5	37	8.0	31	235
Lemon meringue pie, 1/6 of 9" pie	4.3	143	14.0	36	355
Apple pie, 1/6 of 9" pie	4.6	0	18.0	40	405
Cream pie, 1/6 of 9" pie	15.0	8	23.0	46	455
Snacks					
Popcorn, air-popped, 1 cup	tr.	0	tr.	tr.	30
Pretzels, stick, 2¼", 10 pretzels	tr.	0	tr.	tr.	10
Popcorn with oil and salted, 1 cup	0.5	0	3.0	49	55
Corn chips, 1 oz.	1.4	25	9.0	52	155
Potato chips, 1 oz.	2.6	0	10.1	62	147
Pudding					
Gelatin	0.0	0	0.0	0	70
Tapioca, ½ cup	2.3	15	4.0	25	145
Chocolate pudding, ½ cup	2.4	15	4.0	24	150

[1] Total fat = saturated fatty acids plus monounsaturated fatty acids plus polyunsaturated fatty acids.
[2] Percent calories from fat = (total fat calories divided by total calories) multiplied by 100; total fat calories = total fat (grams) multiplied by 9.
oz. = ounce
tr. = trace
Source:
Home and Garden Bulletin. Nutritive Value of Foods. No. 72. United States Department of Agriculture. Human Nutrition Information Service (1986).

Appendix 11: Miscellaneous Fat and Cholesterol Comparison Chart

Product	Saturated Fatty Acids[1] (Grams)	Cholesterol (Milligrams)	Total Fat[1] (Grams)	Calories from Fat[2] (%)	Total Calories
Gravies (½ cup)					
Au jus, canned	0.1	1	0.3	3	80
Turkey, canned	0.7	3	2.5	37	61
Beef, canned	1.4	4	2.8	41	62
Chicken, canned	1.7	3	6.8	65	95
Sauces (½ cup)					
Sweet and sour	tr.	0	0.1	<1	147
Barbecue	0.3	0	2.3	22	94
White	3.2	17	6.7	50	121
Cheese	4.7	26	8.6	50	154
Sour cream	8.5	45	15.1	53	255
Hollandaise	20.9	94	34.1	87	353
Bearnaise	20.9	99	34.1	88	351
Salad Dressings (1 Tablespoon)					
Russian, low calorie	0.1	1	0.7	27	23
French, low calorie	0.1	1	0.9	37	22
Italian, low calorie	0.2	1	1.5	85	16
Thousand Island, low calorie	0.2	2	1.6	59	24
Imitation mayonnaise	0.5	4	2.9	75	35
Thousand Island, regular	0.9	—	5.6	86	59
Italian, regular	1.0	—	7.1	93	69
Russian, regular	1.1	—	7.8	92	76
French, regular	1.5	—	6.4	86	67
Blue cheese	1.5	—	8.0	93	77
Mayonnaise	1.6	8	11.0	100	99

Product	Saturated Fatty Acids (Grams)	Cholesterol (Milligrams)	Total Fat[1] (Grams)	Calories from Fat[2] (%)	Total Calories
Other					
Olives, green, 4 medium	0.2	0	1.5	90	15
Nondairy creamer, powdered, 1 teaspoon	0.7	0	1.0	90	10
Avocado, Florida	5.3	0	27.0	72	340
Pizza, cheese, 1/8 of 15" diameter	4.1	56	9.0	28	290
Quiche lorraine, 1/8 of 8" diameter	23.2	285	48.0	72	600

[1]Total fat = saturated fatty acids plus monounsaturated fatty acids plus polyunsaturated fatty acids.

[2]Percent calories from fat = (total fat calories divided by total calories) multiplied by 100; total fat calories = fat (grams) multiplied by 9.

— = Information not available in the sources used.

Sources:
Composition of Foods: Fats and Oils – Raw • Processed • Prepared, Agriculture Handbook 8-4. United States Department of Agriculture, Science and Education Administration (June 1979).

Composition of Foods: Soups, Sauces, and Gravies – Raw • Processed • Prepared, Agriculture Handbook 8-6. United States Department of Agriculture, Science and Education Administration (February 1980).

Home and Garden Bulletin. Nutritive Value of Foods. No. 72. United States Department of Agriculture. Human Nutrition Information Service (1986).

The First Step in Eating Right is Buying Right
A Guide to Choosing Low-Saturated Fat, Low-Cholesterol Foods

Following a low-saturated fat, low-cholesterol diet is a balancing act: getting the variety of foods necessary to supply the nutrients you need without too much saturated fat and cholesterol or excess calories. One way to assure variety—and with it, a well-balanced diet—is to select foods each day from each of the following food groups. Select different foods from within groups, too, especially foods low in saturated fat (the left column). How many portions and the size of each portion should be adjusted to reach and maintain your desirable weight. As a guide, the recommended daily number of portions is listed for each food group.

	Choose	Go Easy On	Decrease

Meat, Poultry, Fish and Shellfish (up to 6 ounces a day)	*Lean cuts* of meat with fat trimmed, like:
	• beef
	  round, sirloin, chuck, loin
	• lamb
	  leg, arm, loin, rib
	• pork
	  tenderloin, leg (fresh), shoulder (arm or picnic)
	• veal
	  all trimmed cuts except ground
	poultry without skin
	fish
	shellfish
			"Prime" grade
			Fatty cuts of meat, like:
			• beef
			  corned beef brisket, regular ground, short ribs
			• pork
			  spareribs, blade roll, fresh
			goose, domestic duck
			organ meats
			sausage, bacon
			regular luncheon meats
			frankfurters
			caviar, roe

(Cont.)

	Choose	Go Easy On	Decrease
Dairy Products (2 servings a day; 3 servings for women who are pregnant or breastfeeding)	skim milk, 1% milk, low-fat buttermilk, low-fat evaporated or nonfat milk low-fat yogurt low-fat soft cheeses, like cottage, farmer, pot cheeses labeled no more than 2 to 6 grams of fat an ounce	2% milk yogurt part-skim ricotta part-skim or imitation hard cheeses, like part-skim mozzarella "light" cream cheese "light" sour cream	whole milk, like regular, evaporated, condensed cream, half and half, most non-dairy creamers, imitation milk products, whipped cream custard style yogurt whole-milk ricotta neufchatel brie hard cheeses, like swiss, American, mozzarella, feta, cheddar, muenster cream cheese sour cream
Eggs (no more than 3 egg yolks a week)	egg whites cholesterol-free egg substitutes		egg yolks
Fats and Oils (up to 6 to 8 teaspoons a day)	unsaturated vegetable oils: corn, olive, peanut, rapeseed (canola oil), safflower, sesame, soybean margarine; or shortening made from unsaturated fats listed above: liquid, tub, stick, diet	nuts and seeds avocados and olives	butter, coconut oil, palm oil, palm kernel oil, lard, bacon fat margarine or shortening made from saturated fats listed above

(Cont.)

	Choose	Go Easy On	Decrease
Breads, Cereals, Pasta, Rice, Dried Peas and Beans (6 to 11 servings a day)	breads, like white, whole wheat, pumpernickel, and rye breads; pita; bagel; English muffin; sandwich buns; dinner rolls; rice cakes low-fat crackers, like matzo, bread sticks, rye krisp, saltines, zwieback hot cereals, most cold dry cereals pasta, like plain noodles, spaghetti, macaroni any grain rice dried peas and beans, like split peas, black-eyed peas, chick peas, kidney beans, navy beans, lentils, soybeans, soybean curd (tofu)	store-bought pancakes, waffles, biscuits, muffins, cornbread	croissant, butter rolls, sweet rolls, danish pastry, doughnuts most snack crackers, like cheese crackers, butter crackers, those made with saturated oils granola-type cereals made with saturated oils pasta and rice prepared with cream, butter or cheese sauces; egg noodles
Fruits and Vegetables (2 to 4 servings of fruit and 3 to 5 servings of vegetables a day)	fresh, frozen, canned or dried fruits and vegetables		vegetables prepared in butter, cream or sauce

(Cont.)

	Choose	Go Easy On	Decrease	(Cont.)
Sweets and Snacks (avoid too many sweets)	low-fat frozen desserts, like sherbet, sorbet, Italian ice, frozen yogurt, popsicles	frozen desserts, like ice milk	high-fat frozen desserts, like ice cream, frozen tofu	
	low-fat cakes, like angel food cake	homemade cakes, cookies, and pies using unsaturated oils sparingly	high-fat cakes, like most store-bought, pound, and frosted cakes	
	low-fat cookies, like fig bars, gingersnaps	fruit crisps and cobblers	store-bought pies	
	low-fat candy, like jelly beans, hard candy		most store-bought cookies	
	low-fat snacks like plain popcorn, pretzels		most candy, like chocolate bars	
			high-fat snacks, like chips, buttered popcorn	
	nonfat beverages like carbonated drinks, juices, tea coffee		high-fat beverages, like frappes, milkshakes, floats, and eggnogs	

Label Ingredients

Go easy on products that list any fat or oil first or that list many fat and oil ingredients (decrease) and unsaturated ingredients (go easy on). The following lists clue you in to names of saturated fat ingredients.

	carob, cocoa	cocoa butter
	oils, like corn, cottonseed, olive, safflower, sesame, soybean or sunflower oil	animal fat, like bacon, beef, chicken, ham, lamb, meat, pork or turkey fats, butter, lard
	nonfat dry milk, nonfat dry milk solids, skim milk	coconut, coconut oil, palm or palm kernel oil

cream
egg and egg-yolk solids
hardened fat or oil
hydrogenated vegetable oil
milk chocolate
shortening or vegetable shortening
vegetable oil (could be coconut, palm kernel or palm oil)

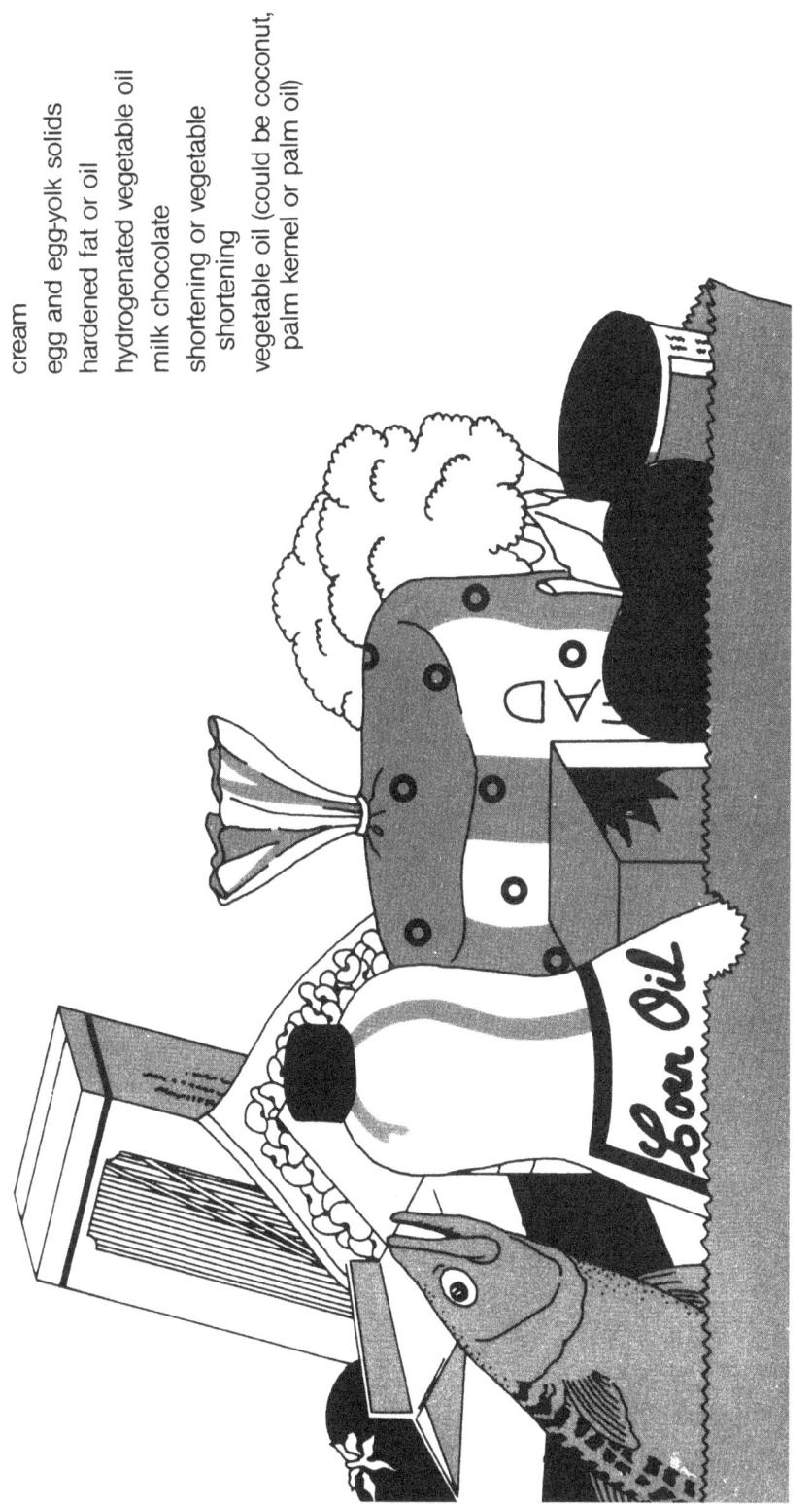

www.ingramcontent.com/pod-product-compliance
Lightning Source LLC
Chambersburg PA
CBHW031243160426
43195CB00009BA/588